THE BIBLE CURE® FOR

HEARTBURN
AND INDIGESTION

DON COLBERT, M.D.

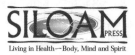

Living in Health—Body, Mind and Spirit

THE BIBLE CURE FOR HEARTBURN AND INDIGESTION
By Don Colbert, M.D.
Published by Siloam Press
A part of Strang Communications Company
600 Rinehart Road
Lake Mary, FL 32746
www.siloampress.com

Scripture quotations marked NKJV are from the
New King James Version of the Bible. Copyright
© 1979, 1980, 1982 by Thomas Nelson, Inc.,
publishers. Used by permission.

Library of Congress Catalog Card Number:
99-93492
International Standard Book Number:
0-88419-651-8

This book is not intended to provide medical advice
or to take the place of medical advice and treatment
from your personal physician. Readers are advised to
consult their own doctors or other qualified health
professionals regarding the treatment of their
medical problems. Neither the publisher nor the
author takes any responsibility for any possible
consequences from any treatment, action or
application of medicine, supplement, herb or
preparation to any person reading or following the
information in this book. If readers are taking
prescription medications, they should consult with
their physicians and not take themselves off of
medicines to start supplementation without the
proper supervision of a physician.

02 03 04 05   12 11 10 9 8
Printed in the United States of America

Preface

There's
Hope for Heartburn
and Indigestion

As uncomfortable and embarrassing as they can be, digestive problems are not life-threatening, and the cures are remarkably simple and easy to take. Yes, they can indicate other more serious medical problems. But, even the most serious problems usually have treatments that are readily available. Often digestive problems and their accompanying symptoms are related to lifestyle and nutrition. The good news is that you can take positive steps to eliminate this discomfort in your life.

In this booklet, you will discover God-given ways in the natural and spiritual that you can take to overcome digestive tract problems. God wills that you walk in divine health so that you can serve and glorify Him. Lay hold to this promise:

"Don't be impressed with your own wisdom. Instead, fear the LORD and turn your back on evil. Then you will gain renewed health and vitality" (Prov. 3:7–8). This Bible Cure booklet is your opportunity to follow God's wisdom in the natural and supernatural, and in doing so, you will gain *renewed health and vitality!*

A mountain of research exists on Americans and their digestive systems. Like anything else, the research can be presented in a lopsided fashion. For example, each year 62 million Americans are diagnosed with a digestive disorder. The incidence and prevalence of most digestive diseases increase with age. But if we stopped here, we would be painting a pretty grim picture. But the truth that is often overlooked by those outside of the medical profession is that there are answers to these 62 million cases.

Look at some of the other facts that are available about digestive problems:

- About 25 million adults suffer daily from heartburn.
- There are more reported cases of women with irritable bowel syndrome (IBS) than there are men with IBS.

- More than 60 million Americans are reported to have experienced gastroesophageal reflux disease (GERD) and heartburn at least once a month.
- Recent studies seem to indicate that GERD in infants and children is more common than previously recognized and may produce recurrent vomiting, coughing and other respiratory problems.

Although all of these reports are accurate, as presented above, they only show one side of the story. The other side is a story of hope, help and healing. Twenty-five million Americans can find relief from heartburn. Sixty million Americans can find help for GERD. Children around the nation can find health and healing. The Bible cure is an excellent place to begin and to find hope.

This Bible Cure booklet is designed to help you keep your body fit and healthy through preventing and eliminating digestive problems. In this booklet, you will

*uncover God's divine plan of health
for body, soul and spirit
through modern medicine, good nutrition
and the medicinal power
of Scripture and prayer.*

This booklet was designed with you in mind. Key Scriptures placed throughout will help you focus on the healing power of God through His Word. These inspiring texts will guide your prayers and direct your thoughts toward God's plan of divine health for you. In this booklet, you will discover how to eliminate heartburn, indigestion, bloating and gas through chapters on:

I am praying that God will give you the understanding and wisdom you need to apply both natural and spiritual means to overcome digestive problems. As you read this book, may you be helped tremendously and encouraged greatly by the Bible cure for digestive problems.

—Don Colbert, M.D.

vii

A BIBLE CURE PRAYER
FOR YOU

Heavenly Father, I know that You are my Creator. I've seen the wonders of Your power and excellence at work in this world and in my body. You truly are an awesome God, and there is none like You in all of creation. You are my Maker, and You have fearfully and wonderfully created my digestive system. Because of Your handiwork, my body will receive all the nutrients it needs for health.

Lord, I submit my life and my health to You and Your Bible cure. By the power of Your Holy Spirit, I ask You to grant me wisdom to apply the truths I learn from the Bible cure. You know my every need, my every situation, every cell of my being, and I am fully persuaded that I can trust You with my very life.

Forgive me when I fall short in regards to the care of my body, which is the temple of Your Holy Spirit. (See 1 Corinthians 6:19.) Help me, Lord, from this point forward, to live in divine health and serve You with my whole spirit, soul and body. Satan has no authority in my life; You are my King. Satan has no power over this body; You are all powerful. I will glorify Your name for Your wondrous grace and Your miraculous powers of refreshing and restoration. Amen.

Chapter 1

Beating Digestive Tract Problems

As the Bible declares, "You made all the delicate, inner parts of my body and knit me together in my mother's womb. Thank you for making me so wonderfully complex! Your workmanship is marvelous—and how well I know it" (Ps. 139:13–14). One of the most remarkable creations of God is your digestive system. How marvelous it is that God both created the fuel and the system to power our physical bodies. The fuel He created is revealed in the beginning of the Bible cure.

God said in Genesis, "Look! I have given you the seed-bearing plants throughout the earth and all the fruit trees for your food. And I have given all the grasses and other green plants to the animals and birds for their food" (vv. 29–30). You are about to discover how some of the plants, herbs, seeds and grasses God created will actually help your digestive system heal!

The digestive tract is one of the most used—and abused—systems in our bodies. Since the digestive tract is responsible for converting the food we eat into the nutrients we need to live, it's only natural that it can be the source of a whole host of ailments. More often than not, we give our digestive tracts poor materials with which to work. Subsequently, diseases of the digestive tract send more people to the hospital in the United States than any other group of disorders. These disorders include hiatal hernia, heartburn, peptic ulcer disease, lactose intolerance, constipation, irritable bowel syndrome, diverticulosis, diverticulitis and more.

> *Don't you realize that all of you together are the temple of God and that the Spirit of God lives in you? God will bring ruin upon anyone who ruins this temple. For God's temple is holy, and you Christians are that temple*
> —1 CORINTHIANS 3:16–17

A popular saying is that we are what we eat. A much truer statement is that we are what we actually digest and absorb. A person can be on a very well-balanced diet and be taking a variety of nutritional supplements, but if he is not adequately absorbing them, then much of the supplements or benefits are simply being wasted.

To understand the digestion and absorption functions of the gastrointestinal (GI) tract, you must first understand how the GI tract functions. Digestion actually begins with signals from the brain that occur when it decides that the body needs food. These signals trigger the digestive tract to begin producing the necessary enzymes and components for digestion.

Eliminate Stress and Negative Emotions Before Eating

I believe it is critically important to ask the blessing prior to eating, since this helps to relax our minds and bodies in preparation for receiving the food. If a person is upset, angry, fearful or has other negative emotions while eating, these negative emotions stimulate the sympathetic nervous system, which in turn causes decreased secretion of hydrochloric acid. This causes decreased secretion of pancreatic enzymes, which makes it harder to digest the food.

Also I believe that food allergies and sensitivities may be the direct result of negative emotions during eating. Before eating, take time to thank God and to meditate on His goodness and provision. As you pray, ask the Holy Spirit to use the nutrients in your food to strengthen you. Claim His promise: "Don't be afraid, for I am with you. Do not be dismayed, for I am your God. I will strengthen you. I will help you. I will uphold you with my victorious right hand" (Isa. 41:10). You may need to take several deep breaths and relax. Release any negative emotions; then, give thanks to the Lord and bless the food.

This process is one of the most important things you can do in order to have good digestion. Paul says in Philippians 4:6–7:

> Do not worry about anything, but in everything by prayer and supplication with thanksgiving, let your requests be made known to God. And the peace of God, which surpasses all understanding, will guard your hearts and your minds in Christ Jesus.
>
> —NKJV

Whatever it is that is causing you to experience these negative emotions—be it frustration, anxiety or stress—God is able, through the avenue of prayer, to move into our lives and speak to those storms, bringing perfect peace. Not only does God give peace to us, the kind of peace that goes beyond our ability to explain and understand, but His peace acts as a barrier around our hearts and minds in order to protect us from future anxieties.

Life in such a stressed-out, high-paced society often forces us to do things that are in direct conflict with healthy lifestyle choices—like eating on the run. As a result, our bodies and minds are not adequately prepared to digest our food. Then along come symptoms of heartburn, indigestion, gas and bloating, and we wonder why. Take time simply to slow down, relax and allow God's peace to clear the mind of negative emotions. Give thanks to God for your

> *And God said, "Look! I have given you the seed-bearing plants throughout the earth and all the fruit trees for your food. And I have given all the grasses and other green plants to the animals and birds for their food." And so it was.*
> —GENESIS 1:29–30

food. This is one of the most important things that you can do to start the process of healthy digestive function.

A BIBLE CURE HEALTH TIP

Before Eating

- Relax and slow down from your stressful pace of life (Ps. 37:7).
- Meditate on God's Word (Ps. 1:1–2).
- Clear your mind of negative emotions thinking on positive ones (Phil. 4:8).
- Pray and give thanks (Phil. 4:6–7).

Chewing Your Food

The next important step in digestion involves chewing the food. Although chewing is an automatic reflex action triggered by the feel of food against the teeth and the inside of the mouth, it is very important that we learn to chew our food thoroughly. Each bite should be chewed approximately twenty to thirty times. As we chew, the food becomes mixed with our saliva. The saliva contains an enzyme called amylase. Think of enzymes as a pair of chemical scissors that take the long starch molecules in our food and begin to chop them up into smaller pieces called simple sugars.

Starches are packed full of energy that our bodies need. But in order to get to that energy, the starches must be broken apart and the energy released. It is this breaking down of starch into simple sugars that allows our bodies to absorb its energy.

For example, you may have noticed before that if you chew on a cracker or piece of bread for long enough, it will eventually begin to taste sweet. This is because the enzymes in your mouth are breaking down the starch into simple sugars.

So what happens to food that goes through our system without being properly digested? Undigested materials clog our intestines and can have toxic effects on our bodies, setting the stage for infections, fatigue and degenerative disease.

Understand How Your Body Digests Food

It's important for you to understand how your body digests food. Without this understanding, you will not know why certain steps are necessary for you to take in order to eliminate heartburn, indigestion, bloating and gas. Allow me to walk you through the basic processes of your digestive system.

The digestive system is a group of organs that work like wrecking equipment to break down the chemical components of food into tiny nutrients that can be absorbed to generate energy for the body. It accomplishes this through the use of digestive juices. As food passes through the body, it is broken down into small units that can be absorbed into the blood and lymph systems. Some units are used for energy, some as building blocks for tissues and cells and some are stored for future or emergency use.

In addition, your digestive system is continuously building and replacing its cells and tissues, which continuously are sluffing off and dying.

The large, hollow organs of the digestive system contain muscles that enable their walls to move. The movement of the organ walls can do two things: propel food and liquid through the organs and mix the contents within each organ. Typical movement of the esophagus, stomach and intestine is called *peristalsis*. The action of peristalsis looks like an ocean wave moving through the muscle. The muscle of the organ produces a narrowing and then propels the narrowed portion slowly down the length of the organ. These waves of narrowing push the food and fluid in front of them through each hollow organ.

This complex operation we call *digestion* begins in the mouth. The mouth and teeth grind the food into small particles. The tongue manipulates the food between the teeth for chewing. Food is chewed, pulped and mixed with saliva to become a soft mass, called *bolus,* which will easily travel down the esophagus. Saliva, which is more than 99 percent water and contains the enzyme amylase (mentioned earlier in this chapter), lubricates chewing and swallowing and begins the process of digestion.

After you have thoroughly chewed your food, it is swallowed by way of the esophagus, entering into your gut region, which consists of the stomach, small intestines, large intestines, rectum and anus. Serious digestion begins in the stomach. The healthy stomach has a pH between 1.5 and 3. This is due to the hydrochloric acid that is secreted by the stomach.

Did you know that the hydrochloric acid in your stomach is strong enough to burn a hole through carpet and to melt the iron in a nail? This powerful acid is part of God's incredible design to help soften the food and to kill any germs it may contain. The reason that hydrochloric acid doesn't eat a hole through your stomach is because God lined your stomach with mucus. Not only that, but your stomach lining is actually replaced every three days to insure its strength and usefulness!

The stomach is like a giant sack that connects the esophagus and the duodenum (the first part of the small intestine). At the junction of the esophagus and stomach, there is a ring-like valve, called the *esophageal sphincter,* closing the passage between the two organs.

However, as the food approaches the closed ring, the surrounding muscles relax and allow the food to pass. If not closed properly after the food enters, the acidic contents of the stomach can move up into the esophagus and cause a burning sensation (heartburn).

> *You must never eat any fat or blood. This is a permanent law for you and all your descendants, wherever they may live.*
> —LEVITICUS 3:17

The stomach consists of layers of muscle and nerves that continue the breakdown of food that was begun in the mouth. It is also a storage compartment, which enables us to eat only two or three meals a day. If this weren't possible, we would have to eat about every twenty minutes. The average adult stomach stretches to hold from two to three pints and produces approximately the same amount of gastric juices every twenty-four hours.

The stomach has several functions:

- It's a storage bin, holding a meal in the upper portion and releasing it a little at a time into the lower portion for processing.
- It's a blender. The strong muscles contract and mash the food into a sticky, slushy mass (called *chyme*).
- It's a sterilizing system. The cells in the stomach produce hydrochloric acid that kills germs in food.
- It's a digestive tub. The stomach produces digestive fluid (which contains the enzyme pepsin), that breaks down the chemicals in food so that they can be distributed as fuel for the body.

The sight, smell or taste of food triggers the process of digestion, so that the stomach is prepared when the food arrives. Every time you get a whiff of your favorite foods or see a commercial that makes your mouth water, the body begins a digestive process. This processing of the food in the stomach usually takes between one to four hours, but different foods take different lengths of time to digest: starches stay in the stomach one to two hours; proteins stay three to five hours, and fats stay more than five hours. The end result of this process is a semi-liquid food termed chyme.

Next, the food moves into the small intestine. If the small intestine were not looped back and forth upon itself, it could not fit into the abdominal space it occupies. It measures eighteen to twenty-three feet in the average adult, which makes it about four times longer than the person is tall. It is about as big around as a paper towel tube and is divided into three sections:

- The *duodenum,* a receiving area for chemicals and partially digested food from the stomach
- The *jejunum,* where most of the nutrients are absorbed into the blood
- The *ileum,* where the remaining nutrients are absorbed before moving into the large intestine.

The intestines process about 2.5 gallons of food,

liquids and bodily waste every day. In order for enough nutrients to be absorbed into the body, they must come in contact with large numbers of intestinal cells. Each of these cells contains thousands of tiny finger-like projections called "villi." Villi line the wall of the small intestines. In one square inch of small intestine, there are about 20,000 villi. The villi sway constantly to stir up liquefied food and remove the nutrients. These smaller particles that have been broken down are able to pass into the villi and are taken up by very small capillaries, where they are then carried to the liver.

The muscles which encircle the small intestine constrict about seven to twelve times a minute to move the food back and forth, to churn it, knead it and to mix it with gastric juices. The small intestine also makes waves that move the food forward, but these are

If you will listen carefully to the voice of the LORD your God and do what is right in his sight, obeying his commands and laws, then I will not make you suffer the diseases I sent on the Egyptians; for I am the LORD who heals you.
—EXODUS 15:26

usually too weak and infrequent to allow the food

to stay in one place until the nutrients can be absorbed. If a toxic substance enters the small intestine, these movements may be strong and rapid to expel the poisons quickly.

Finally, all of the digested nutrients are absorbed through the intestinal walls. Minerals are absorbed mainly in the duodenum; carbohydrates, proteins and water soluble vitamins are absorbed mainly in the jejunum. Fats and fat-soluble vitamins are absorbed in the ileum. The waste products of this process are propelled into the colon, where they remain, usually for a day or two, until the feces are expelled by a bowel movement.

The large intestine, or colon, is laid out in the gut like a squared version of a question mark. The last few inches of the colon make up the rectum, which is a storage site for solid waste. This waste leaves the body by way of an external opening called the anus. Not all that we eat can be digested, so the waste must be disposed of in an efficient way.

Substances that have not been absorbed while in the small intestine enter the large intestine in the form of liquid and fiber. The large intestine, or bowel, is sometimes called the "garbage dump" of the body, because the materials that reach it are of very small use to the body and are sent on from absorbs fluids and recycles them into the blood stream. The second half condenses the wastes into feces and secretes mucus, which binds the substances and lubricates it to protect the colon and ease its passage. Of the two to two and one-half gallons of food and liquids taken in by the average adult, only about twelve ounces of waste enters the large intestine. Feces is comprised of about three quarters water. The remainder is protein, fat, undigested food roughage, dried digestive juices, cells shed by the intestine and dead bacteria.

✓ A BIBLE CURE HEALTHFACT

You should have a bowel movement at least every fourteen hours. A typical timetable for digestion is as follows:

- 0 hours—start eating
- ½ hour—stomach is full
- 2 hours—chyme entering duodenum
- 6 hours—stomach nearly empty
- 12 hours—nutrients being absorbed in the small intestine
- 18 hours—wastes are forming in the large intestine
- 24 hours—feces are ready to leave the body

Ideally, if you eat three large meals a day, you should have three bowel movements a day because God has designed our bodies to process food at a very consistent pace. Unfortunately, our diets tend to keep our bowel movements from being regular. For instance, high-fat diets will take much longer than necessary to move through our system. Thirty to thirty-five grams of fiber a day is essential for maintaining a healthy colon. Fiber helps to move food through the colon faster. People with sedentary lifestyles need to increase both their fiber intake and exercise in order to help their digestive processes work more efficiently. We will talk more about dietary guidelines and digestive problems (like constipation) of the colon and intestines in chapter five.

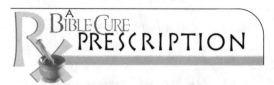

BIBLE CURE
PRESCRIPTION

Beginning Steps for
Beating Digestive Problems

Check which steps you will begin to take right now:

❑ Pray, relax and reduce stress

❑ Chew food slowly

❑ Focus on God and clear my mind of negative emotions

❑ Review how my digestive system works

Chapter 2

Beating Common Causes of Heartburn and Indigestion

We know in Scripture that Timothy had problems with his digestive tract and Paul actually gave him some practical advice. (See 1 Timothy 5:23.) Just as God cared about Timothy's stomach, He also cares about every detail of our lives, even how we digest food. As the psalmist reveals, "You watched me as I was being formed in utter seclusion, as I was woven together in the dark of the womb. You saw me before I was born. Every day of my life was recorded in your book. Every moment was laid out before a single day had passed" (Ps. 139:15–16).

The God who made you will also heal you and show you how to walk in divine health. Let's explore some ways that God has provided for your heartburn and indigestion to be healed.

Now that you understand the basic functions of the gastrointestinal (GI) tract, we can discuss causes and solutions for heartburn, indigestion, bloating and gas. There are many different causes for heartburn and indigestion, which include hiatal hernia, GE reflux, gastritis, ulcer disease, gallbladder disease, excessive acid production, low acid production, pancreatic insufficiency and food allergy.

The Problem of Decreased Gastric Acid Secretion

I believe one of the most common causes of heartburn and indigestion is hypochlorhydria, which is decreased gastric acid secretion or, more simply put, not enough hydrochloric acid. Approximately 50 percent of people over the age of fifty have low stomach acidity.

The stressful lifestyles of most Americans account for much of this. Is your body telling you that you are under too much stress? Place an x beside each of the items in the following box that are true for you:

❑ Difficulty falling asleep
❑ Not rested when you get up from sleeping
❑ Physical aches and pains
❑ Depressed or anxious
❑ Panic feelings, including your heart racing
   and perhaps feeling light-headed
❑ Stomach upset
❑ Diarrhea

If you checked four or more of the previous items, you may be experiencing too much stress. You might take the following stress test just to measure how stressed you may be right now. If you score high and are having gastrointestinal problems, then in all probability too much stress is one of the precipitating factors.

How Stressed Are You?
Your Stress Scale

In the following table you can look up representative changes in your life and see how much stress value each of these changes is adding to your life. Note any item that you may have experienced in the last twelve months. Then, total up your score.

STRESS EVENT	VALUES

1. Death of Spouse 100
2. Divorce 60
3. Menopause 60
4. Separation from living partner 60
5. Jail term or probation 60
6. Death of close family member other
   than spouse 60
7. Serious personal injury or illness 45
8. Marriage or establishing life partnership 45
9. Fired at work 45
10. Marital or relationship reconciliation 40
11. Retirement 40
12. Change in health of immediate family member .40
13. Work more than 40 hours per week 35
14. Pregnancy or causing pregnancy 35
15. Sex difficulties 35
16. Gain of new family member 35
17. Business or work role change 35
18. Change in financial state 35
19. Death of a close friend (not a family member) .30
20. Change in number of arguments
    with spouse or life partner 30
21. Mortgage or loan for a major purpose 25
22. Foreclosure of mortgage or loan 25
23. Sleep less than 8 hours per night 25

21

24. Change in responsibilities at work 25
25. Trouble with in-laws or with children 25
26. Outstanding personal achievement 25
27. Spouse begins or stops work 20
28. Begin or end school .20
29. Change in living conditions (visitors in the
    home, change in roommates,
    remodeling house) 20
30. Change in personal habits
    (diet, exercise, smoking) 20
31. Chronic allergies 20
32. Trouble with boss 20
33. Change in work hours or conditions 15
34. Moving to new residence 15
35. Presently in pre-menstrual period 15
36. Change in schools 15
37. Change in religious activities 15
38. Change in social activities
    (more or less than before) 15
39. Minor financial loan .10
40. Change in frequency of family get-togethers . . .10
41. Vacation 10
42. Presently in winter holiday season 10
43. Minor violation of the law 5

TOTAL SCORE:_____

I have asked you to look at the last twelve months of changes in your life. This may surprise you. It is crucial to understand that a major change in your life has effects that carry over for long periods of time. It is like dropping a rock into a pond. After the initial splash, you will experience ripples of stress. And these ripples may continue in your life for at least a year.

So, if you have experienced total stress within the last twelve months of 250 or greater, even with normal stress tolerance, you may be overstressed. Persons with low stress tolerance may be over-stressed at levels as low as 150.[1]

Overstress Will Make You Sick

Carrying too heavy a stress load is like running your car engine past the red line, or leaving your toaster stuck in the "on" position; or running a nuclear reactor past maximum permissible power. Sooner or later, something will break, burn up or melt down. What breaks depends on where the weak links are in your physical body. And this is largely an inherited characteristic.

So to recap, stress can cause a lot of problems for your body, one of which is low stomach acidity—which in turn can cause heartburn and indigestion. Stress can turn a healthy body into an unhealthy body very quickly. It's no coincidence that the Bible deals with the issue of stress more than 250 times, approaching the subject from the aspect of its cure—peace.

Jesus said, "Peace I leave with you; my peace I give you. I do not give to you as the world gives. Do not let your hearts be troubled and do not be afraid." That's quite a

> *You must serve only the LORD your God. If you do, I will bless you with food and water, and I will keep you healthy.*
> —Exodus 23:25

promise—one well worth meditating on and remembering daily.

Your Nervous System and Digestive Tract

Let's take a look at your nervous system and how it may affect your digestive tract. The nervous system is composed of two branches: the sympathetic and the parasympathetic.

The sympathetic nervous system is one of the branches of the autonomic nervous system. When stimulated, the sympathetic nervous system causes an increase in heart rate and a rise in blood pressure. Then the pupils become dilated. Blood is shunted away from the GI tract and shunted to the muscles in order to empower them for fighting or fleeing. As a result, when these nerves are stimulated, there is increased peristalsis (rhythmic muscle movement) in the small intestines and in the colon, often causing a person to eliminate his bowel contents so that he can run faster.

The other arm to the autonomic nervous system is the parasympathetic response. In the parasympathetic response, there is a slowing of the heartbeat, a constriction of the pupils and a stimulation of certain digestive glands. The parasympathetic response is ideal for digestion. However, this response only occurs when you are relaxed and calm. Due to our fast-paced society, most people work, live and eat in a sympathetic dominant state. This is similar to driving your car all the time with your accelerator to the floor.

Eventually these people become exhausted due to the continual drain on the adrenal hormones. In a sympathetic dominance, blood flow is shunted away from the digestive tract, and there is a decrease in hydrochloric acid secretion. Therefore, digestion suffers dramatically.

Type A Personalities

Most people who are type A personalities (which means they are impatient, tense, highly driven and highly aggressive) are usually deficient in hydrochloric acid and thus more prone to heartburn and indigestion.

The sad thing is that they are treating this with antacids such as Maalox, Mylanta, Tums, Rolaids, Zantac and Tagamet. Actually, these compound the problem by lowering the acid even more rather than helping a person. They only made you feel better. Due to the low secretion of hydrochloric acid, there is a decrease in the release of pancreatic enzymes since hydrochloric acid turns on the release of the pancreatic enzymes.

> *Praise the LORD, I tell myself; with my whole heart, I will praise his holy name. Praise the LORD, I tell myself, and never forget the good things he does for me. He forgives all my sins and heals all my diseases.*
> —PSALM 103:1–3

A deficiency of hydrochloric acid will, in turn, cause a deficiency in pancreatic enzymes. This, in turn, causes incomplete digestion of proteins, fats and carbohydrates. This, in turn, leads to fermentation of incompletely digested carbohydrates, putrefaction of incompletely digested proteins and rancidity of incompletely digested fats.

Whatever is not adequately digested and absorbed in the GI tract can become toxic due the effects that bacteria, yeast or parasites may have on the food. In other words, if the bacteria, yeast or parasites get to the food before we are able to digest it and assimilate it, they can ferment the carbohydrates, producing excessive gas. They can putrefy the protein which releases very toxic materials and rancifies the fats.

Of course, there is a cure for the problems caused by a sympathetic dominant, type A personality. It's the Bible cure, and it's called the Sabbath. Once a week, our bodies need a chance to rest. This spiritual law has tremendous physical benefits, allowing our bodies to rest, refresh and renew. There are also steps that we can take throughout the day in order to give our bodies some mini-Sabbaths.

Steps to Take Before Eating

In correcting low stomach acid output, I believe first you must learn how to relax prior to eating.

Keep in mind that relaxation techniques are no different than dieting or exercise. These are simply proven methods for bringing our bodies under submission to our spirit and to God's will. Paul said, "I beat my body and make it my slave so that after I have preached to others, I myself will not be disqualified for the prize" (1 Cor. 9:27, NIV). Paul didn't mean that he physically beat his body. Rather, he stayed in shape through exercise and self-control.

Relaxation exercise

Learn how to relax with simple exercises such as a progressive relaxation tape. Lie down in a comfortable setting with soothing praise and worship music; beginning with the toes, flex the toes for just a second or two, then relax. Then flex the ankles for a second or two, then relax. Go through every muscle group flexing and then relaxing, all the way through your face muscles. This will put the body in a very relaxed state.

Deep breathing

Maybe you need a technique that can be completed in less time than the progressive relaxation technique listed above. Instead, practice deep breathing by simply lying down with a book on the abdomen, taking a deep breath in and watching the book rise in the air. Then exhale. Do this five to ten times, and it will also reduce the stress. Practice abdominal breathing rather than chest breathing in order to relax.

A brisk walk

You may also want to go on a brisk walk prior to eating. This seems to relax many people. Also you can

> *For God has not given us a spirit of fear and timidity, but of power, love, and self-discipline.*
> —2 Timothy 1:7

meditate on the Word of God or read scriptures aloud to help you relax. Isaiah 26:3 says, "You will keep in perfect peace all who trust in you, whose thoughts are fixed on you!" By being in a relaxed state you will avoid the "fight-or-flight" sympathetic response, which greatly interferes with digestion.

Drink water

I recommend strongly that you drink one to two glasses of filtered or distilled water thirty minutes prior to each meal. We have a mucous layer that covers the lining of the stomach. The mucous layer is to prevent the hydrochloric acid from burning the stomach. We would self-digest our own stomachs if it were not for the mucous layer.

In order for the mucous layer to be adequate, we need adequate hydration. That is why it is critically important to drink one to two glasses of water thirty minutes before each meal. I recommend a minimum of two quarts of water a day.

If you do have symptoms of chronic heartburn and indigestion, I recommend seeing a nutritional doctor prior to starting the nutritional program. Your nutritional doctor must determine first if your stomach produces inadequate amounts of hydrochloric acid. He may do this with nutritional testing.

Also, your physician should rule out an ulcer or gastritis, since hydrochloric acid would aggravate these conditions.

In order to correct low gastric acid secretion you should start by taking six hundred milligrams of hydrochloric acid at each large meal. If it is a small meal, you should have only three hundred milligrams of HCL. The dose should be gradually increased under the direction of your nutritional doctor.

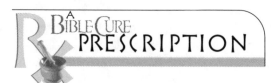

Preventing Heartburn

How will you relax before a meal?

_____

_____

How many glasses of water will you drink daily?

_____

What steps do you plan to take to reduce your stress?

_____

Write a prayer thanking God for your food and living water. Also ask Him to guide you in finding new ways to rest and relax.

_____

_____

_____

_____

Chapter 3

Beating Indigestion Problems

How often has the pleasure of eating a good meal been ruined for you by painful heartburn? I have wonderful news: You no longer have to endure these problems! It's possible with God's guidance and your own self-control to beat indigestion problems and feel good. Let's explore in greater depth some simple ways you can relieve heartburn through diet, relaxation, exercise and losing weight.

It all begins with your mental attitude and spiritual outlook. Start by replacing negativity with thanksgiving. Decide to act rather than sit back and suffer. Find a friend who will encourage you in taking the steps mentioned in this chapter. And pray for strength to follow through. Remember,

God is not merely a healer; He is your Healer. The Bible says, "If you will listen carefully to the voice of the LORD your God and do what is right in his sight, obeying his commands and laws, then I will not make you suffer the diseases I sent on the Egyptians; for I am the LORD who heals you" (Exod. 15:26).

Hiatal Hernias

One major cause of heartburn and indigestion is hiatal hernia. While surgery may be recommended by your physician, there are some steps you can take to relieve the symptoms and possibly avoid the need for surgery.

A hiatal hernia simply is a small portion of the stomach pouching out above the diaphragm. This is usually due to pregnancy, obesity and increased abdominal pressure. Approximately 50 percent of people over the age of fifty have hiatal hernias. However, only 5 percent of these with hiatal hernias actually experience esophageal (GE) reflux.

I believe the best treatment for both hiatal hernias and GE reflux is to lose weight, especially in the abdominal area.

Keys for Weight Loss

1. Drink two quarts of filtered or bottled water a day. It is best to drink two 8-ounce glasses, 30 minutes before each meal, or one to two 8-ounce glasses 2½ hours after each meal.
2. Thirty minutes of brisk walking four times a week.
3. You may eat fruit; however, avoid fruit juices.
4. Things to avoid:
   - sugar
   - alcohol
   - all fried foods
   - starches (breads, crackers, bagels, potatoes, pasta, rice, corn, black, pinto, red beans.) Also limit your intake of bananas.
5. Eat these foods:
   - fresh fruit
   - steamed, stir-fried or raw vegetables
   - lean meats
   - salads, preferably with extra-virgin olive oil and vinegar
   - nuts (almonds, organic peanuts) and seeds

6. Take fiber supplements such as Fiber Plus, Perdiem Fiber or any other fiber without NutraSweet or sugar.
7. Take 2 tablespoons of Milk of Magnesia each day if constipated.
8. Follow the diet suggested throughout this booklet.
9. For snacks, choose Iron Man PR Bars, Zone Bars or Balance Bars. My favorite snack bar is the yogurt honey peanut balance bars. These may be purchased from my office or at a health food store.
10. Do not eat past 7 P.M.

Coping With
Reflux Esophagitus

Reflux esophagitus is caused by the stomach acid refluxing up into the esophagus which occurs when the valve (the esophageal sphincter) does not close properly. The reason why this valve usually doesn't close properly is due to diet.

What Stimulates Reflux Esophagitus?

Take this simple self-test to see if you are avoiding those foods and fluids that often trigger reflux esophagitus. The following list includes what you need to avoid. Check those items that you will begin avoiding today!

- ❑ Chocolate
- ❑ Coffee
- ❑ Alcohol
- ❑ High-fat foods
- ❑ Drinking excessive fluids with a meal (It is very important not to drink over four ounces of fluid with each meal, since excess fluid will increase tendencies to have reflux if the valve is not functioning properly.)

Avoid Chilled Liquids
With Your Meals

Indigestion is extremely common in the United States. One of the main reasons why Americans get frequent indigestion is because we drink cold liquids with our meals. First I recommend that you drink approximately one or two 8-ounce glasses thirty minutes prior to eating. Preferably it should be room temperature water. During meals, limit your intake of fluid to approximately four ounces of fluid. These drinks should also be room temperature.

Drinking ice cold liquids with a meal slows down digestion. It would be like trying to start a fire, while dumping water on the fire just as it starts to get hot. So it is with our digestion. By continually drinking cold fluids with our meals we wash out many of our digestive juices, and we significantly slow down the process of digestion.

> *Words satisfy the soul as food satisfies the stomach; the right words on a person's lips bring satisfaction. Those who love to talk will experience the consequences, for the tongue can kill or nourish life.*
> —PROVERBS 18:20–21

Take a Chewable Calcium Tablet

Calcium, in the form of a chewable calcium tablet such as Tums, is able to make the valve close. Chew a calcium tablet such as a Tums immediately after each meal and take a chewable calcium tablet at bedtime.

More Steps You Can Take . . .

Elevate the head of your bed. If heartburn or reflux esophagitus are still not relieved, I recommend that you place a four inch concrete block under the bedpost at the head of your bed. This will allow gravity to prevent the flow of hydrochloric acid up the esophagus. Take DGL. I recommend that you take DGL, which is a special form of licorice. Take two chewable tablets thirty minutes before each meal and at bedtime.

Drink aloe vera juice. I recommend drinking ½ quart to 1 quart throughout your day. Avoid drinking too much, however. It can lead to diarrhea.

One of the real keys to eliminating digestive problems to beating indigestion problems is by carefully monitoring what we eat and by losing weight. I know that losing weight is more than just a physical issue. It's so important that you seek God's help to overcome any tendencies you have to overeat.

Remember the promise of Scripture, "For I can do everything with the help of Christ who gives me the strength I need" (Phil. 4:13).

Take These
Spiritual Steps Right Now

- Ask God to break any food addiction or eat disorder that afflicts you.
- Seek the Spirit's guidance for selecting someone to help hold you accountable for your eating habits.
- Ask God's Spirit to reveal to you the foods you need to avoid and the right foods for your system to digest.
- Accept God's desire and provision to supply all your needs, including your physical needs for food.

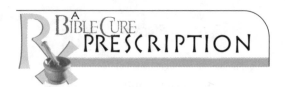

Reducing Weight

Losing weight is essential for reducing digestive problems. Complete the following sentences:

One reason it's hard for me to lose weight is

_____.

The first step I will take to lose weight is

_____.

A friend who will encourage me as I lose weight is

_____.

As I lose weight, I will pray and meditate about

_____.

The form of exercise I will do regularly is

_____.

The one food that I need God's strength to avoid eating is

_____.

Chapter 4

Beating Pancreatic Insufficiency, Ulcers and Gastritis

We need God's knowledge for understanding how the awesome organs of our complex bodies work for our good health. We are so wonderfully made, and God has provided specific instructions to care for every organ in the body. Our Maker desires for us to be in good health.

In fact, we need others to join with us and help us pray for our health. The apostle John set the example when he wrote, "Dear friend, I am praying that all is well with you and that your body is as healthy as I know your soul is" (3 John 2). As you learn about your body and decide to take care of it, claim God's healing prayer with others for divine health by agreeing with one another in prayer.

Lay hold to this marvelous promise from God: "I also tell you this: If two of you agree down here on earth concerning anything you ask, my Father in heaven will do it for you" (Matt. 18:19).

The Pancreas

One very important organ for which we need to know how to care is the pancreas. The pancreas is a digestive organ in the abdomen that's located just below the stomach. Its primary job is

> *Anything you eat passes through the stomach and then goes out of the body. But evil words come from an evil heart and defile the person who says them.*
> —MATTHEW 15:17–18

to produce enzymes that break down food for digestion and absorption. Each day the pancreas secretes about 1.5 quarts of pancreatic juice into the small intestine. Enzymes secreted include lipases, which digest fat, proteases, which digest proteins, and amylases, which digest starch molecules. The primary characteristics of pancreatic insufficiency are impaired digestion, malabsorption, nutrient deficiencies and abdominal discomfort.

You can take positive steps to help your pancreas

digest food and assist your entire digestive system in processing what you eat so that you will feel better and eliminate many uncomfortable symptoms.

You can overcome pancreatic insufficiency and other digestive problems by taking some simple Bible cure steps. Don't be discouraged. The uncomfortable symptoms you are having should be checked by a physician, but they can be overcome with lifestyle and nutritional changes. Let's explore some basic steps you can take.

Pancreatic Insufficiency

One of the most common causes of abdominal bloating and gas that I have found has been pancreatic insufficiency.

Examine your stools. A fairly simple way to determine if you have pancreatic insufficiency is to look at your stools. We look at our food as it goes in our mouth, but we never look at it when it comes out. If you are passing undigested food in the stool, there is a very strong likelihood that you are suffering pancreatic insufficiency. This is fairly common in elderly people.

Use pancreatic enzymes. The treatment for pancreatic insufficiency is simply pancreatic

43

enzymes. I recommend pancreatin, which contains amylase, lipase and protease. Also, I prefer a full-strength pancreatic extract rather than the low-potency products. I prefer the nonenteric-coated products. If you are a vegetarian, you may take bromelain and papain, which come from pineapple and papaya.

Ulcers and Gastritis

Common causes of indigestion are ulcers and gastritis. Stomach acid is highly acidic. So if you have a thin layer of mucous covering the stomach lining, then you will be predisposed to forming an ulcer, especially if you are taking an anti-inflammatory medicine, aspirin or alcohol.

Drink lots of water. I believe adequate hydration—three quarts a day, preferably two 8-ounce glasses, thirty minutes before each meal—is the most important thing in preventing ulcer disease. Mucus is mostly water. Since it is the mucus lining of the stomach that protects the stomach from ulcers, it stands to reason that poor hydration will eventually take its toll on the mucus production in the stomach.

Avoid irritants. Equally important is avoiding

alcohol, aspirin and non-steroidal anti-inflamma-tory drugs (such as Advil, Motrin and Aleve). These drugs also thin out the mucus lining in the stomach, making room for ulcers and gastritis.

Lower your stress. As we discussed in chapter two, it is critically important that you decrease your stress.

Peptic Ulcer Disease

H. pylori is a bacteria that is commonly associated with peptic ulcer disease. Factors that predispose one to developing *H. pylori* include low output of hydrochloric acid, an inadequate mucous layer protecting the stomach and low antioxidant status of the stomach lining. Smoking is also harmful in that it overstimulates acid secretion.

Things to Avoid or Decrease

If you have an ulcer, it is critical that you change your lifestyle. Avoid alcohol, aspirin and other an-tiinflammatories. Stop smoking and decrease or avoid caffeinated beverages.

Drink a lot of water. You should increase your water intake to at least two to three quarts a day.

Drink fresh juice. Cabbage juice is excellent

for healing ulcers, but you should have at least a quart a day.

Take DGL tablets. DGL, which is a special form of licorice, is extremely important in helping to heal and to protect you from further ulcer formation. You should take DGL—two chewable 380 milligram tablets approximately thirty minutes before each meal and at bedtime.

Drink aloe vera juice. Aloe vera juice is also helpful in preventing and treating ulcer disease. You need to drink approximately ½ to 1 quart of aloe juice throughout the day. Avoid excessive amounts that may cause diarrhea.

Take glutamine. The amino acid glutamine in a dose of 500–1000 milligrams, taken thirty minutes prior to each meal, is also helpful in preventing or treating ulcer disease.

Take gamma-oryzanol. Gamma-oryzanol comes from brown rice and contains powerful antioxidants that are able to heal ulcers. These include ulcers of the stomach and the duodenum, which is the first part of the small intestines. Gamma-oryzanol is also found in rice bran, rice bran oil or in capsule form. You should take 100 milligrams, three times a day, about ten minutes before your meals.

Take a special form of bismuth. If you have *H-pylori,* which is the bacteria that usually causes ulcers, you need to take a special form of bismuth called bismuth subcitrate. This substance can be prescribed by your nutritional doctor and is taken in a dose of 240 milligrams two times a day before meals. There is a simple blood test that can be performed by your physician in order to determine if you do have this bacteria. There are also different antibiotic treatments which may be prescribed by your physician.[1]

Overcoming Food Intolerances

Food intolerances, often called food allergies, commonly produce GI symptoms which include indigestion, gas, bloating, diarrhea, spastic colon and malabsorption, to mention but a few. Other conditions commonly associated with food allergies include eczema, asthma, frequent ear infections, sinusitis and fatigue.

Consuming certain foods excessively may increase our sensitivities to them and thus increase the possibility of allergic reactions. While it is possible to become sensitive or allergic to almost any food, certain frequent offenders include milk, eggs, wheat, corn and chocolate.

Quite often people have only approximately ten foods that they eat on a continual basis, so they need to expand the variety of foods they eat.

Variety is the spice of life, and this goes for our food also. It is important to eat a different type of food on a daily basis so that you will not develop food allergies.

Patients with food allergies commonly have a low output of hydrochloric acid from their stomachs. Also they secrete insufficient amounts of pancreatic enzymes, especially the proteases. The proteases are enzymes that break down proteins. Your food must be thoroughly chewed, then be acted upon by hydrochloric acid. If proteins are not completely digested, then any other leftover protein should be broken down by proteases secreted by the pancreas. If the protein is not broken down adequately into amino acids and short chain peptides, the large protein molecule can actually produce an allergic response.

This occurs when the large protein crosses (usually between the intestinal villi) into the bloodstream to be absorbed. This can thus lead to four different types of allergic-type reactions:

1. Hives may break out all over the body.
2. The airway may become constricted.
3. Wheezing may occur.
4. A delayed hypersensitivity reaction may occur hours to days after consuming the food. Symptoms may include malabsorption, diarrhea, gas, bloating, eczema, fatigue.

There is no simple cure for food allergies. I believe that basic treatment for food allergies involves a good nutritional program by a nutritional doctor, which includes adequate amounts of HCL, pepsin and pancreatic enzymes. You may follow a low antigenic diet where you stop eating the foods that you normally eat on a daily basis and begin eating foods that rarely produce allergies.

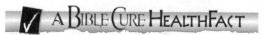

A BIBLE CURE HEALTHFACT

**Foods That Rarely
Produce Allergies**

- Rice
- Turkey
- Bananas
- Chicken
- Potatoes
- Apples

Food rotation is extremely important in preventing food allergies. Each food in the diet is consumed only one day out of every four days. For example, you may eat chicken for lunch and dinner on Tuesday, which is fine. But rotate your foods so you don't eat chicken again until Saturday at the earliest. This decreases the chance of a food allergy from each of the foods. It also makes it much easier to isolate foods, which cause allergic reactions.

A BIBLE CURE HEALTH TIP

The Coca Pulse Test

Perform the Coca Pulse Test. Take your pulse for one minute prior to eating. Then place a bite of the food to which you might be allergic on your tongue. After thirty seconds, recheck your pulse. If the pulse rate goes up over six beats per minute you may be sensitive or allergic to the food. The higher the pulse goes up, usually the more severe the allergy or sensitivity.

Combining Your Foods

Proper food combining may also help you with digestive problems including heart burn, indigestion, gas and bloating. If you have normal GI function, you do not necessarily need to follow this program. In food combining, fruits are always eaten alone because they are much more easily digested than other foods.

Protein foods such as meats and milk products should not be eaten with starches such as breads, pasta, potatoes, beans and rice. Vegetables such as broccoli, asparagus and lettuce, can be combined with either starches, such as bread pasta, potatoes, or with protein foods, such as meats and milk products.

The logic for this food combining is that

> *So I tell you, don't worry about everyday life whether you have enough food, drink, and clothes. Doesn't life consist of more than food and clothing? Look at the birds. They don't need to plant or harvest or put food in barns because your heavenly Father feeds them. And you are far more valuable to him than they are.*
> —MATTHEW 6:25–26

for optimal digestion starches need an alkaline environment, whereas proteins need an acidic environment. When these two types of food are eaten together they interfere with one another, therefore causing digestion that is incomplete and which takes much longer than normal. Therefore, many proteins and starches remain undigested, resulting in proteins putrefying in the small intestines while carbohydrates ferment, producing bloating and gas.

I personally have developed severe food sensitivities. My food sensitivities were resolved finally after desensitizing through the N.A.E.T. method of desensitization. To find a physician in your area who is certified in this technique, go to the Internet Web site: www.naet.com. It is still critically important to have adequate hydrochloric acid, pepsin and pancreatic enzyme, even after one has desensitized.

> *Don't worry about anything; instead, pray about everything. Tell God what you need, and thank him for all he has done. If you do this, you will experience God's peace, which is far more wonderful than the human mind can understand. His peace will guard your hearts and minds as you live in Christ Jesus.*
> —PHILIPPIANS 4:6–7

I know that taking the steps I have outlined in this chapter may not be easy. Certain foods that we may be allergic to will be tempting. But God can help you avoid eating what will irritate your digestive system. He is also able to heal any problem you may have with pancreatic insufficiency, ulcers or gastritis. I want to encourage you to pray for your healing and to invite the spiritual leaders in your church to pray for you. Confidently believe this promise:

> Are any among you sick? They should call for the elders of the church and have them pray over them, anointing them with oil in the name of the Lord. And their prayer offered in faith will heal the sick, and the Lord will make them well. And anyone who has committed sins will be forgiven. Confess your sins to each other and pray for each other so that you may be healed. The earnest prayer of a righteous person has great power and wonderful results.
> —JAMES 5:14–16

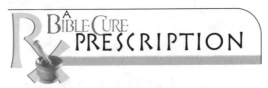

BIBLE CURE
PRESCRIPTION

**Overcoming Pancreatic Insufficiency,
Ulcers and Gastritis**

If you have pancreatic insufficiency, check the
steps you will take:

❑ Check your stools, and consult your physician.

❑ Use pancreatic enzymes.

If you have food allergies, describe how you will:
Combine your foods

_____

Use supplements

_____

Drink adequate fluids

_____

Avoid foods to which you are allergic

_____

Ask others to pray for you

_____

Chapter 5

Beating Digestive Problems in the Colon and Intestines

G od has created important substances, partic-
ular foods with fiber, which can help our intestines and colon stay healthy. You may be telling
others how poorly you feel. Know that your com-
plaints will not help you heal either physically or
spiritually. However, you can begin to speak life
and confess God as your Healer right now.
Proverbs declares, "A person's words can be life-
giving water; words of true wisdom are as refreshing as a bubbling brook" (Prov. 18:4).

Many digestive problems originate with the bacteria that live in our colons. The bacteria actually
serve some very useful purposes except when those
bacteria become excessive. The number of bacteria in the large bowel or colon is usually about

one hundred trillion. We may have as much as three to five pounds of bacterial mass living in our colons. In our colon the bacteria function actually to synthesize different vitamins, break down toxins and prevent overgrowth of dangerous bacteria such as shigella and salmonella. The majority of our immune system is actually located in the lining of our small intestines.

The problem with bacteria occurs when there are bacteria and yeast overgrowth in the small intestines. This is a common problem and results, usually, in the overuse of antibiotics and inadequate amounts of hydrochloric acid secretion. When bacterial and yeast overgrowth occur in the small intestines, excessive gas and bloating result. Often, this results from the fermentation of the sugars in starch (potatoes, bread, corn, pasta) and simple sugar (cakes, pies, candies, cookies).

Bacteria in the small intestine can also putrefy proteins, producing strong chemicals that can damage the lining of the small intestines. This can result in a condition called a leaky gut. A leaky gut in turn can lead to more food allergies, diarrhea, bloating, gas and abdominal pain.

If you have an overgrowth of yeast in the small intestine, there is a much higher chance that you'll have parasites in the small intestines, since this condition creates a perfect breeding ground for parasites.

In order to determine if you do have overgrowth of bacteria in the small bowel, you should have a comprehensive stool analysis along with a breath test; this test will reveal if there are high amounts of hydrogen in the breath, which would signify bacterial overgrowth. These tests can be performed by a nutritional doctor in your area. To find a nutritional doctor in your area who is able to perform these tests, call the Great Smokey's Lab at (800) 522-4762.

Although the idea of bacteria and parasites invading our digestive system sounds pretty alarming, remember that the treatment and cure for these things is remarkably simple and easy. Were it not for God's incredible design of our bodies, this might not be true. However, since these problems are relatively common, it is reassuring that they can be easily remedied through natural methods.

Bacterial Overgrowth

Overgrowth of bacteria in the small intestines eventually will destroy the enzymes that line the surface of the intestinal cells, thus leading to inadequate digestion and absorption of carbohydrates and sugars. This leads to more fermentation and more bloating, gas and possibly diarrhea.

Patients with overgrowth of bacteria and yeast in the small intestines usually have excessive mucous production by the cells that line the intestines. Unlike the stomach in which mucous is useful, this thick layer of mucous prevents contact between the enzymes in the intestinal cells and the disaccharides, which are double sugars such as lactose (or milk sugar), sucrose (which is cane sugar), maltose, and iso-maltose (which is corn syrup as in many candies).

> *I know how to live on almost nothing or with everything. I have learned the secret of living in every situation, whether it is with a full stomach or empty, with plenty or little. For I can do everything with the help of Christ who gives me the strength I need.*
> —PHILIPPIANS 4:12–13

Simple sugars such as glucose, fructose and galactose do not need to be enzymatically split in order to be transported from the intestines into the blood stream. However, double sugars have to be split by enzymes in the intestinal lining in order to be absorbed. But since the mucous lining is so thick, the enzymatic reaction with the double sugar cannot take place. Thus, the sugars are left to ferment in the small intestines leading to more gas, bloating and diarrhea.

Steps to Take

Add enzymes. If you do have bacterial overgrowth, first you should be on adequate amounts of hydrochloric acid, pepsin and pancreatic enzymes. Follow a very low-carbohydrate diet that excludes sugar, milk products and excessive amounts of starchy foods.

Reduce certain starches and sugars. Refined sugar exhausts the pancreas, which produces insulin, and increases the chance of gallstones. Patients with bacterial overgrowth in the small intestines are unable to tolerate certain starches since it leads to increased fermentation. These starches include almost any cereal grain, including wheat, oats, corn, rye, rice, millet that has been made into bread, crackers, cereal, pasta, flour, pizza, cookies.

The carbohydrates in these grains are

fermented by bacteria and yeast in the small intestines. The only carbohydrates that are allowed are the carbohydrates found in fruits, lactose-free yogurt, honey, and vegetables such as salads, celery, cucumbers, asparagus, onions and carrots. You may eat also most nuts, except for peanuts. However, if you are not able to tolerate nuts, and they cause diarrhea, they should be stopped. Avoid all foods made with white, refined, sugar.

Avoid potatoes. Avoid eating both sweet potatoes and regular potatoes, along with most all beans, including soybeans.

Avoid most all juices. Also avoid all fruits that are canned with syrup. Drink water or water with a squeeze of lemon. Drink organic apple cider in small amounts.

Avoid certain foods. Foods that usually cause the most gas and bloating are milk products and all products made with white sugar. Avoid alcohol and especially beer.

I believe this diet is the mainstay of treatment for bacterial and yeast overgrowth. In addition, you need adequate amounts of hydrochloric acid, pepsin and pancreatic enzymes.

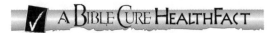

Beating Constipation

Bloating and gas are also commonly due to constipation. Most likely, this is the most common gastrointestinal disorder and is due usually to insufficient intake of water. Intake of water should be at least two to three quarts a day. Also it is due to insufficient fiber intake, which should normally be 25–35 grams of fiber per day.

HEALTHFACT HEALTHFACT HEALTHFACT HEALTHFACT HEALTHFACT HEALTHFACT HEALTHFACT

The Importance of Fiber

Fiber protects us from many diseases and is critically important to our digestive processes. Fiber is also very important in treating people with overgrowth of bacteria and yeast in the small intestine. Insoluble fiber does not feed the bacteria, and is not fermented rapidly in the small intestine. Also it helps to bind and inactivate many toxins in the intestines.

I believe the best insoluble fiber is microcrystaline cellulose. Some patients do well with rice bran, which contains gamma-oryzanol. This is a powerful antioxidant that helps to heal both stomach and intestinal ulcerations.

How to Eat More Fiber

To get adequate fiber in your diet, follow the U.S. Department of Agriculture's Food Guide Pyramid, which recommends the following:[1]

- Eat 2–4 servings of fruit.
- Eat 3–5 servings of vegetables.
- Eat 6–11 servings of cereal and grain foods each day. (Make sure they are whole grain.)
- Begin your day by eating a whole-grain cereal that contains at least 5 grams of fiber per serving.
- Try to eat vegetables raw as much as possible, as cooking may reduce fiber content.
- Try not to peel fruits (such as apples and pears) and vegetables, because much of the fiber is found in the skin.
- Add beans to soups, stews and salads.
- Eat fresh and dried fruits as snacks.
- Read food labels for fiber content.

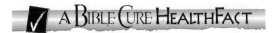
What Does Fiber Do?

Fiber is an important part of a healthy diet, because it aids normal bowel function and help maintain regularity. When part of a diet low in saturated fat and cholesterol, fiber has been associated with a reduced risk of certain cancers, diabetes, digestive disorders and heart disease.

Foods high in soluble fiber include:

- Oat bran
- Oatmeal
- Rice bran
- Barley
- Beans
- Peas
- Citrus fruits

Foods high in insoluble fiber include:

- Whole-wheat breads
- Wheat cereals
- Rye
- Barley
- Carrots
- Wheat bran
- Whole-grain rice
- Cabbage
- Brussels sprouts

You should also take in *lactobacillus aci-dophilus* and *lactobacillus bifidus*. Lactobacillus acidophilus is a friendly organism that helps the body fight disease and restore health. Modern research has discovered that acidophilus kills the harmful bacteria strain of *E. coli* in the intestinal tract. Acidophilus also breaks milk sugar down into lactic acid. Bacteria that produce putrefaction and gas in the intestines cannot live in lactic acid. Acidophilus also has the unique ability to help the body in the production of the B vitamins in the system.

This is especially helpful since there are a lot of common agents which destroy B vitamins. A few are antibiotics, birth control pills, sugar and refined foods and coffee. Acidophilus inhibit the growth of pathogenic bacteria and inhibit many of the chemicals these bad bacteria produce. They also prevent altered intestinal permeability.

You need at least three billion organisms of bifido bacteria and lactobacillus per day. Acidophilus grows mainly in the small intestines, whereas lactobacillus grows well in the large intestines.[2]

Use Herbs

Herbs also help to kill abnormal bacteria, yeast and parasites in the small intestine. Herbs that are used commonly to do this include oregano in a dose of five tablets, three times a day with meals, and garlic in a dose of 500 milligrams, one tablet, three times a day with meals. Sometimes I need to add the medication nystatin, 500,000 units per tablet, one tablet, three times a day along with the oregano and garlic in order to decrease the population of yeast in the small intestines.

Finally, aerobic exercise such as brisk walking, cycling and swimming, for twenty to thirty minutes, three to four times a week is very important in preventing constipation.

There are many forms of fiber you can take that include psyllium, oat bran, rice bran, flaxseeds ground into a powder, pectin and guar gum. I also strongly advise my patients to take a drink that is high in chlorophyll which includes wheat grass, barley grass, alfalfa and the different algae, which include blue-green algae, spiralina and chlorella. These high chlorophyll foods help to cleanse the colon and prevent constipation.

A BIBLE CURE RECIPE

DR. COLBERT'S DAILY MILKSHAKE

Take a scoop of Divine Health Greens Detox Drink, which contains a mixture of each of the following chlorophyll foods. Either mix thoroughly with orange juice or blend it until smooth and creamy. Drink this mixture on a daily basis.

- Alfalfa
- Barley grass
- Chlorella
- Wheat grass
- Spirulina
- Blue-green algae

Divine Health Nutritional Products may be ordered from the information provided at the back of this book. I drink this concoction as soon as I wake up in the morning, along with freshly squeezed orange juice. I also take it in the evening as soon as I get home from work.

Avoid the Use of Laxatives

Avoid using both herbal laxatives and over-the-counter laxatives, since this can lead to a dependence on the laxative. A healthy, natural laxative that anyone can take is magnesium; it can be taken in the form of magnesium citrate, magnesium glycinate and magnesium aspartate.

Magnesium in a dose of 400 milligrams, three or more times a day will assure most anyone of a regular bowel movement daily. A common magnesium product that will help you feel better is milk of magnesia. Take according to the label instructions.

Never suppress the urge to have a bowel movement, since this is commonly associated with constipation. Also eliminate processed foods such as white bread, white flour, white noodles, white rice and any other processed food. It usually takes two to three times as long to pass processed food as it does to pass whole grain foods.

Taking lactobacillus acidophilus and bifidus, approximately three billion colony-forming units a day, is extremely important for patients with constipation. White bread has all of the bran and germ removed during processing, along with approximately 80 percent of the nutrients and virtually all of the fiber. The flour is bleached, which destroys even more vitamins. Next, sugar and hydrogenated fats are added, along with manufactured vitamins.

Make sure to eliminate products such as white bread, which is pure starch without the fiber and nutritional value of whole grain breads. If you add water to white bread, it forms a sticky gluelike substance. Is there any wonder why this food takes double the amount of time to be eliminated from the body? I believe this is one of the main reasons we have so much colon cancer in the U.S. It is the number three cancer killer for both men and women.

Years ago Dr. Dennis Burkitt compared the stools of rural Africans on a fiber-rich diet of over 100 grams of fiber a day with British naval officers who ate mainly meats, white flour and sugar. The Africans had large effortless stools in approximately eighteen to thirty-six hours. In comparison, the British naval officers experienced small, difficult, compact stools in seventy-two to one hundred hours.

Also, the naval officers developed hemorrhoids, anal fissures, varicose veins, diverticulitis, diverticulosis, thrombophlebitus, gallbladder disease, appendicitis, hiatal hernia, irritable bowel syndrome, obesity, high cholesterol, coronary artery disease, high blood pressure, diabetes, hypoglycemia, colon polyps, colon and rectal cancers. The rural Africans only experienced these conditions and diseases when they converted to a

British diet consisting mainly of meats, white flour and sugar. The moral of this story is simply this: Fiber is important and essential for healthy digestion of your food.[3]

Take time right now to pray about your intestinal problems. Your prayers can open you spiritually and physically to God's healing power. He is sending forth His word at this moment to heal you. Claim this Bible cure promise: "He spoke, and they were healed—snatched from the door of death" (Ps. 107:20). Begin praying this:

A BIBLE CURE PRAYER FOR YOU

Almighty God, thank You for my digestive system. Speak Your healing word to my intestines and colon. Help me stay on track in my diet so that I eat the fiber and other foods I need for physically healing. Thank You, Lord, for healing me. Amen.

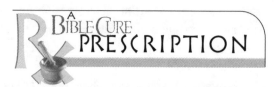

A BIBLE CURE PRESCRIPTION

Overcoming Digestive Problems in the Colon and Intestines

Describe what foods you will eat for adequate fiber intake:

_____

_____

Summarize why you need fiber in your daily diet:

_____

_____

If constipation is a problem, what steps will you take?

_____

Write a prayer for your healing:

_____

_____

_____

_____

Chapter 6

Beating Digestive Problems With Detoxification

Toxins attack both our bodies and spirit. In order to detoxify spiritually, we must repent and ask God's forgiveness. Toxins also abound in the natural order as our bodies are attacked and we must fight off toxic substances and chemicals. It's just as important to be free spiritually of toxins as it is to detoxify spiritually. In fact, spiritual toxins—sin, negative attitudes and emotions, addictions and destructive behaviors—can keep our digestive systems in turmoil. To deal with spiritual toxins, we must detoxify through:

- Confessing sin
- Repenting and turning away from sin
- Asking God's forgiveness

- Receiving His forgiving grace through Christ
- Being committed not to sin again

After spiritual detoxification, physical detoxification also can have wonderful physical benefits. Clinical detoxification is very important in controlling heartburn, indigestion, bloating and gas. I am not talking about detoxification for alcohol or drugs. I am talking about removing toxins that are produced in the body in the intestines and from the environment.

For example, toxins produced within the body include the waste products of cellular metabolism. Cellular metabolism uses nutrients in the presence of oxygen to form energy. An analogy of this is like a log in a fireplace. When a log is burning in the presence of oxygen, smoke is produced. In cellular metabolism, the nutrients used in the presence of oxygen do not produce smoke, but instead they produce cellular debris and free radicals. These waste products of cellular metabolism need to be flushed out of the body on a regular basis. Metabolism may also be impaired due to nutritional deficiencies such as vitamin and mineral deficiencies and excessive stress.

Also toxins are produced within the intestines. Food allergies, food sensitivities, and food intolerance can result in impaired digestion and absorption. As a result the unabsorbed, undigested food actually becomes a toxic material as it leads to putrefaction, fermentation and rancidity.

In addition, bacterial overgrowth, yeast overgrowth or parasitic infections in the small intestine can turn food into toxic metabolites, which are absorbed into the blood stream and can lead to fatigue drowsiness, stupor, muscle aches and cloudy thinking.

Toxins are all around us. Pollutants are in our air and in our water. In addition to these toxins, much of our food is polluted due to pesticides, herbicides, antibiotics and hormones. We live in a toxic world. However, I believe the majority of our toxins are actually produced within our bodies and within our intestines.

Heavy metals are a major source of toxins, especially mercury which comes from fish and from silver fillings in our teeth. Mercury has antibiotic-type affects that kill our good bacteria. As a result, pathogenic bacteria can begin residing in our small intestines; as a result, an overgrowth of yeast and parasites may occur.

One of the best methods of detoxification involves replacing the processed foods that we eat with super foods, which provide essential nutrients and aid in the elimination of toxic material. The simplest of super foods include a high chlorophyll drink first thing in the morning upon awakening, and a detoxification shake for breakfast. For the first week it would be good to drink the detox shake for lunch and dinner. The detox shake will aid in intestinal detoxification and elimination, as well as help support the liver.

As soon as I awaken in the morning I take a super food that is a combination of wheat grass, barley grass, alfalfa, spiralina, chlorella and blue-green algae. This is my own greens detoxification drink. I take this with either orange juice or grapefruit juice and nine chlorella capsules. I then get ready for work. (I described this shake in chapter 5.)

About thirty to forty-five minutes later, I will prepare my detox shake. I take two cups of filtered water and add five teaspoons of freshly ground flaxseeds, which have been ground in a coffee grinder. Then, I add a cup of fresh fruit which may include bananas, strawberries or peaches. I add two tablespoons of flaxseed oil and two tablespoons of granular lecithin. Next I add a teaspoon of lactobacillus acidophilus and bifidus.

Finally, I add two large scoops of a special hypoallergenic protein mixture, which is balanced and does not cause bloating and gas. I use either Ultraclear from Metagenics or Nutraclear from Biotics. You may also use a few drops of liquid Stevia to sweeten. Blend for one or two minutes, then allow to sit for five to ten minutes. I drink approximately half of it for breakfast and the remainder of it throughout the morning. This gives me tremendous energy. It keeps me satisfied throughout the entire morning so that I don't crave food.

Under the care of your own nutritional doctor, you can go on this program for one week, taking the greens detox drink upon awakening in the morning and the detox shake for breakfast, lunch and dinner. This is one of the best detox nutritional programs that I have used. Also, you should also drink at least two quarts of water during the day while on this detox program. Make sure that you get plenty of rest.

If you are very toxic, you may have symptoms of irritability and fatigue as well as nausea or flu-like symptoms. Again, make sure that you are under the care of your nutritional doctor while undergoing this detox program. While going through detoxification, take these steps:

- Avoid meat, eggs, dairy foods, seafood, grains, beans, nuts, seeds, processed foods, fried and refined foods, sweets, coffee, tea, alcohol, spices such as pepper and salt.
- Exercise with brisk walking on a daily basis.
- Take the supplements recommended by your nutritional doctor. This may include hydrochloric acid and pepsin, pancreatic enzymes, beet juice extract for the gallbladder and to thin the bile secretions, milk thistle for detoxifying the liver, drainage formulas for the kidneys, supplements of garlic and oregano to rid the small intestines of yeast, bacteria and parasites.
- During the first week of clinical detoxification you may experience side effects of nausea, diarrhea, constipation, bloating, gas, abdominal pain, indigestion or fatigue. If this persists after a week, it probably indicates a food allergy or an intolerance or sensitivity to either one of the supplements or one of the detoxification foods.

Therefore, you should perform the

Cocoa Pulse Test, in which you take your pulse for one minute and then puts one of your detoxification supplements or foods on your tongue for thirty seconds, rechecking the pulse. If the pulse goes up over six beats, you are probably allergic or sensitive to the detoxification food or supplement. Again, this should be under the direction of a nutritional doctor who has experience and expertise in detoxification. Personally I use this detoxification program on a daily basis at least five days a week. I find that it keeps my body trim and energetic. I have no indigestion, bloating or gas. Also it keeps my mind sharp and prevents the low blood sugar reactions, which I encountered frequently in the past.

By following these simple nutritional pearls, you, too, can be free from heartburn, indigestion, bloating and gas. And remember to detoxify spiritually. The steps I gave you at the beginning of the chapter will help you experience God's peace that will relax you and help you rest. Claim this promise: "But if we confess our sins to him, he is faithful and just to forgive us and to cleanse us from every wrong" (1 John 1:9).

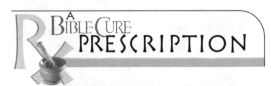

**Overcoming Digestive Problems
With Detoxification**

What steps will you take to detoxify?

_____

_____

Which foods will you avoid?

_____

_____

When will you talk with a nutritional doctor and use detoxification as a regular part of your lifestyle?

_____

_____

What steps do you need to take to detoxify spiritually?

_____

_____

_____

A BIBLE CURE PRAYER
FOR YOU

Almighty God, I thank You that You have proven Yourself to be faithful and merciful to me over and over in my life. I thank You that there is nothing that concerns me that is too great or too small for Your loving care. Even the very hairs on my head are numbered by You. Thank You for providing wisdom and answers to help me overcome digestive problems through natural methods.

In addition, I know that You are My Healer, the God who heals me, as the Word of God says. In the name of Jesus, I boldly declare that this discomfort and pain is finished in my life. In the name of Jesus, I receive the healing power of God at this very moment. I thank You, Lord, that Your healing anointing is flowing through my digestive system right now, strengthening it, calming it, cleansing it and healing it. I receive Your healing power for any ulcers or defects in my digestive tract. I praise You, Lord Jesus, that Your name is greater than every pain and ailment. In the mighty name of Jesus Christ, I declare that I am healed! Amen. I thank You, and I praise You, because You are an awesome heavenly Father. Amen.

A PERSONAL NOTE

From Don and Mary Colbert

God desires to heal you of disease. His Word is full of promises that confirm His love for you and His desire to give you His abundant life. His desire includes more than physical health for you; He wants to make you whole in your mind and spirit as well through a personal relationship with His Son, Jesus Christ.

If you haven't met my best friend, Jesus, I would like to take this opportunity to introduce Him to you. It is very simple.

If you are ready to let Him come into your heart and become your best friend, just bow your head and sincerely pray this prayer from your heart:

Lord Jesus, I want to know You as my Savior and Lord. I believe You are the Son of God and that You died for my sins. I also believe You were raised from the dead and now sit at the right hand of the Father praying for me. I ask You to forgive me for my sins and change my heart so that I can

be Your child and live with You eternally.
Thank You for Your peace. Help me to
walk with You so that I can begin to know
You as my best friend and my Lord. Amen.

If you have prayed this prayer, we rejoice with you in your decision and your new relationship with Jesus. Please contact us at pray4me@strang.com so that we can send you some materials that will help you become established in your relationship with the Lord. You have just made the most important decision of your life. We look forward to hearing from you.

Notes

PREFACE
THERE'S HOPE FOR HEARTBURN AND INDIGESTION

1. Roy E. Palmer, Ph.D., "Gastroesophageal Reflux," *The Daily Apple,* June 1999. Statistics based on "Heartburn may increase your risk of cancer of the esophagus" *The New England Journal of Medicine* (1999): 340:825 831.

CHAPTER 2
BEATING COMMON CAUSES OF
HEARTBURN AND INDIGESTION

1. Adapted from the "Social Readjustment Rating Scale" by Thomas Holmes and Richard Rahe. This scale was first published in the *Journal of Psychosomatic Research,* (1967): vol. II, 214.

CHAPTER 4
BEATING PANCREATIC INSUFFICIENCY,
ULCERS AND GASTRITIS

1. M. Murray Pizzoino, *Encyclopedia of Natural Medicine* (Roctilin, CA: Prima Health, 1998), 814.

CHAPTER 5
BEATING DIGESTIVE PROBLEMS IN THE
COLON AND INTESTINES

1. American Medical Society, Health Insight www.amaassn.org/insight, June 1999.
2. For more information read *The Yeast Connection: A*

Medical Breakthrough by Dr. William G. Crook (Vintage Books, 1986).

3. Summarized from Denis P. Burkitt & Peter A. James, *The Lancet,* July 21, 1973.

Don Colbert, M.D., was born in Tupelo, Mississippi. He attended Oral Roberts School of Medicine in Tulsa, Oklahoma, where he received a bachelor of science degree in biology in addition to his degree in medicine. Dr. Colbert completed his internship and residency with Florida Hospital in Orlando, Florida. He is board certified in family practice and has received extensive training in nutritional medicine.

If you would like more
information about natural and
divine healing, or information about
Divine Health Nutritional Products®,
you may contact
Dr. Colbert at:

DR. DON COLBERT

1908 Boothe Circle
Longwood, FL 32750
Telephone: 407-331-7007
(For ordering products only)

Dr. Colbert's website is
www.drcolbert.com.